DR. SHEILA GRESETH

Top 5 Natural Hacks for Diabetes

Discover Simple Ways to Holistically Improve Blood Sugars Including Tips on Intermittent Fasting, Exercise, and Dietary Dos and Don'ts

This book was professionally typeset on Reedsy.
Find out more at reedsy.com

To my beloved mom, grandpa, and all my diabetic patients,
This dedication is a tribute to your unwavering strength, resilience, and
courage in facing the challenges that diabetes brings.
With love and heartfelt gratitude,
Sheila

Contents

1

Introduction

Diabetes is characterized by the elevation of blood sugars which is a chronic lifelong disease. Diabetes affects 1 out of 11 people in the world and can lead to devastating health complications if left untreated including eye disease, kidney disease, cardiovascular (heart) disease, cerebrovascular disease, peripheral neuropathy (nerve pain), along with many other complication risks. The literal meaning of diabetes mellitus comes from the Greek word diabetes meaning "to pass through" and the Latin word mellitus meaning "sweet." Diabetes is a disease where sugar (sweet) passes through your urine. With the increasing obesity epidemic, 1 in 11 adults have diabetes and approximately 90% of all diabetes is type 2.

I have a passion for preventing diabetes, but I work in the thick of treating diabetes every day. My background began as an Intensive Care Registered Nurse caring for the extremely ill and progressed to my current clinical practice as a Nurse Practitioner in Endocrinology. I graduated with my Doctorate of Nursing Practice in 2017 and began my journey as a hormone specialist. Approximately 80-90% of my practice is treating ALL types of diabetes.

My hope for this book is to provide simple steps that can be implemented for any individual trying to prevent or heal their body naturally from the dangers of ANY type of diabetes.

Of note, it is very important to work with your current provider when implementing lifestyle modifications as these can lead to the reduction or elimination of medications such as insulin.

In "Top 5 Natural Hacks for Diabetes" we will explore 5 topics that can make a tremendous impact in improving your overall quality of life but also controlling your diabetes/glucose levels. These topics include Fasting, Exercise, Low glycemic foods, Foods to avoid, and glucose-balancing supplements and herbs.

2

Intermittent Fasting

As many of us know there is a craze about intermittent fasting, but why? Let's dig into this. When done correctly fasting can provide numerous health benefits and can be sustained lifelong, unlike other fad diets. Historically, our ancestors hundreds of years ago naturally practiced intermittent fasting, this is how our bodies were made to work. We didn't have refrigerators or pantries full of food to access upon waking, people had to hunt and gather food in the morning and would break their fast after the work was complete. Breakfast does not have to be an early morning meal, the word originated from the first meal of the day that "breaks" your "fast".

The common saying "Breakfast is the most important meal of the day" is correct, but when and how you break your fast is the important part. The typical breakfast food we think of today may include cereal, donuts, pastries, pancakes, and waffles. As many can see, these are foods extremely high in carbohydrates, preservatives, and sugars which then start our day out on the wrong foot.

Intermittent fasting is not a one-size-fits-all but should be individualized for each person. In this chapter, I will guide you through a simple plan that fits you and a few of the benefits!

Let's get started!

So why on earth would someone want to intermittent fast? Some of the benefits of intermittent fasting include:

1. **Weight loss**: Intermittent fasting can help facilitate weight loss by promoting a calorie deficit. By restricting the time window for eating, individuals may naturally consume fewer calories, leading to weight loss over time.

2. **Improved insulin sensitivity**: Intermittent fasting has been shown to improve insulin sensitivity, which is crucial for regulating blood sugar levels. This can help lower the risk of type 2 diabetes and metabolic syndrome.

3. **Enhanced metabolic health**: IF may lead to improvements in various markers of metabolic health, including blood pressure, cholesterol levels, and triglycerides. These improvements can reduce the risk of heart disease and other chronic conditions.

4. **Autophagy**: Intermittent fasting can trigger autophagy, a cellular process that involves the removal of damaged or dysfunctional cells and components. This process may help protect against age-related diseases and promote cellular repair and renewal.

5. **Brain health**: Some studies suggest that intermittent fasting may have neuroprotective effects and could potentially reduce the risk of neurodegenerative diseases like Alzheimer's and Parkinson's disease. It may also improve cognitive function and mood.

6. **Longevity**: Emerging research in animals and some human studies suggests that intermittent fasting may extend lifespan and promote longevity by reducing oxidative stress and inflammation in the

body.

7. **Simplicity and flexibility**: Intermittent fasting is relatively simple to implement and can be adapted to fit individual preferences and lifestyles. It doesn't require special foods or supplements, making it a convenient approach for many people.

Now that you know the benefits and why intermittent fasting is important to not only promote health but also its healing powers, let's dig into what this may look like for you.

The prevalent misunderstanding revolves around the timing of breaking your fast. While many advocate for completing a 16-18 hour fast, studies indicate that benefits start manifesting even within a 10-16 hour fasting period. Some individuals opt for extended fasting during the day, followed by a condensed eating window in the afternoon or evening spanning 4-8 hours. For instance, a 4-hour eating window could involve fasting until 3:00 pm and consuming meals until 7:00 pm, effectively bypassing what's typically considered breakfast. I propose a different approach, explaining its potential efficacy. A knowledgeable naturopath, Barbara O'Neill, often advises: "Eat breakfast like a king, lunch like a queen, and supper like a pauper."

Breakfast is your most important meal and should be the most nutritious, packed with fiber, proteins, healthy fats, and minimal carbohydrates. The question is, "When should I have my breakfast?" Here is what a typical/ideal day of eating looks like for me:

- 5 AM: Wake up
- 10-11 AM: Breakfast (Eat like a king)
- 2-3 PM: Lunch (Eat like a queen)
- 5-6 PM: Supper (Eat like a pauper)

- 9-10 PM: Bedtime

This schedule allows for approximately a 16-18 hour fast every day. However, the key to success and making this a sustainable lifestyle change lies in the food choices that are made at each meal.

If you work nights, you can adapt this schedule by swapping AM times for PM times. For instance, if you wake up at 7 PM, this plan can still work for you—just adjust the times to suit your needs and those of your family. Here are three simple tips to help anyone succeed with intermittent fasting long-term:

1. **Start Slow**: If you frequently snack or eat late, begin by reducing these habits before adopting a plan like the one above. For example, start by eliminating all eating after supper. Then, minimize or stop snacking between meals to allow your gut to fully digest your food and prepare for the next meal.
2. **Keep Meal Times 3-4 Hours Apart**: Digestion typically takes around 3-4 hours, so spacing your meals accordingly can help with this process.
3. **Eat Breakfast Like a King, Lunch Like a Queen, and Supper Like a Pauper**: Prioritize nutritious, substantial meals in the morning and lighter meals in the evening.

When able you should eat all your foods in this order 1. Fiber 2. Protein (plant proteins are superior to animal protein) 3. Healthy fats 4. Carbohydrates last. This ensures that your blood sugars do not spike as high or fall too quickly from a high amount of sugar or carbohydrate. Check out the section in Chapter 3 for Healthy Meal Recipe Ideas.

Remember, one size does not fit all. Use this information to create a plan that works best for you.

3

Exercise

Starting an exercise routine can feel overwhelming due to busy schedules, health issues, and limited access to equipment, among other factors. A main goal for many with exercise is to assist in weight loss, but the broader health benefits of exercise far surpass its role in weight management. I want to share simple routines and ideas to help you overcome these obstacles and incorporate daily exercise into your life.

High-Intensity Interval Training (HIIT) is an excellent way to maximize the benefits of exercise in a short amount of time. Most of the advantages of HIIT can be achieved in as little as 15 minutes. HIIT involves short bursts of intense effort, typically at over 75% of your maximal power, followed by brief periods of rest or low-intensity recovery.

To gain health benefits from HIIT, you should engage in high-intensity activity for 30 seconds, pushing yourself as hard as possible. This is followed by a recovery period, which varies based on your current fitness level. The recovery period can range from 1-2 minutes to over 15 minutes, depending on how quickly your heart rate recovers. These intervals should be repeated six times.

The Benefits of HIIT

Improves Insulin Sensitivity

HIIT workouts have been shown to significantly enhance insulin sensitivity. This means that the body becomes more efficient at utilizing glucose from the bloodstream, thereby lowering blood sugar levels and reducing the risk of insulin resistance and type 2 diabetes. Moreover, increased insulin sensitivity can lead to enhanced energy levels, enhanced fat metabolism, better weight management, and improved glucose levels. By incorporating HIIT into a fitness regimen, individuals not only boost their cardiovascular health and endurance but also optimize their body's ability to regulate blood sugar levels, promoting long-term wellness and vitality.

Improves Mood/Mental Health

Engaging in HIIT can have a profound impact on mood, particularly for individuals with diabetes. Regular HIIT sessions stimulate the release of endorphins, often referred to as the body's natural "feel-good" chemicals, which can help alleviate stress, anxiety, and depression commonly associated with managing diabetes.

Additionally, HIIT workouts promote increased blood flow to the brain, enhancing cognitive function and overall mental well-being. For those with diabetes, who may face additional emotional challenges due to the demands of blood sugar management, the mood-boosting effects of HIIT can provide much-needed relief and a sense of empowerment. Furthermore, the sense of accomplishment and progress that comes with completing challenging HIIT sessions can bolster confidence and resilience, further improving overall mood and quality of life. Integrating HIIT into a diabetes management plan not only benefits physical health but also contributes to a more positive and resilient mindset.

Decreases Body Fat

Research on HIIT and its efficacy in reducing body fat has shown promising results. Numerous studies have demonstrated that HIIT is highly effective in promoting fat loss, often surpassing traditional moderate-intensity continuous training (MICT) in terms of efficiency. For example, a meta-analysis published in the British Journal of Sports Medicine found that HIIT was associated with significantly greater reductions in total body fat percentage compared to MICT, with an average decrease of 1.5% body fat after just 12 weeks of HIIT. Furthermore, HIIT has been shown to target visceral fat, the type of fat that accumulates around organs and is linked to an increased risk of chronic diseases such as diabetes and cardiovascular disease. Research indicates that HIIT can lead to a notable reduction in visceral fat, with one study reporting a decrease of up to 17% in visceral fat volume following a 12-week HIIT program.

Additionally, HIIT's post-exercise calorie burn, known as excess post-exercise oxygen consumption (EPOC) or the "afterburn effect," contributes to its effectiveness in reducing body fat. HIIT workouts elevate the metabolic rate and increase oxygen consumption for hours after exercise, leading to greater calorie expenditure even during periods of rest. This phenomenon has been supported by research, with studies showing that HIIT can elevate post-exercise metabolism by up to 9% compared to traditional steady-state exercise. Overall, the combination of HIIT's ability to enhance fat oxidation during exercise and its potent metabolic effects post-exercise makes it a highly efficient strategy for reducing body fat and improving body composition.

Increase Strength and Endurance

HIIT stands out as an effective method for boosting both strength and endurance concurrently. By incorporating short bursts of intense exercise interspersed with brief recovery periods, HIIT engages various muscle groups while challenging the cardiovascular system. This dual focus prompts adaptations that lead to significant improvements in both strength and endurance over time. HIIT's high-intensity nature stimulates muscle fibers to grow stronger and more resilient, contributing to enhanced strength. Moreover, repeated exposure to intense efforts improves the body's ability to sustain prolonged activity, thereby augmenting endurance. Research findings consistently support the efficacy of HIIT in enhancing both strength and endurance.

Example HIIT routines (15 min daily)

Depending on your fitness level the rest period may differ, take the time needed to recover even if this is 10+ minutes.

NO EQUIPMENT HIIT WORKOUT
   Warm-up (3 minutes):

1. Jumping Jacks - 1 minute
2. Arm Circles (30 seconds forward, 30 seconds backward)
3. Jog in Place - 1 minute

Main Workout (15 minutes):

Perform each exercise for 30-40 seconds at high intensity, followed by 1-2 minutes of rest before moving on to the next exercise. Be creative and use any combination of the exercises below to complete 6 exercises total.

1) Burpees:

- Start in a standing position.
- Drop down into a squat position with your hands on the floor.
- Kick your feet back into a push-up position.
- Perform a push-up (optional).
- Jump your feet back to the squat position.
- Explode up into a jump, reaching your arms overhead.

2) Mountain Climbers:

- Start in a plank position with your hands directly under your shoulders.
- Drive one knee toward your chest, then quickly switch legs.
- Continue alternating legs at a rapid pace.

3) Jumping Lunges:

- Start in a lunge position with your right leg forward and left leg back.
- Jump up explosively, switching legs mid-air.
- Land with your left leg forward and right leg back.
- Repeat, alternating legs with each jump.

4) Push-ups:

- Start in a plank position with your hands slightly wider than shoulder-width apart.

- Lower your body until your chest nearly touches the floor.
- Push through your palms to return to the starting position.
- Modify by dropping to your knees if needed.

5) Squat Jumps:

- Start in a squat position with feet shoulder-width apart.
- Explosively jump up, extending your legs fully.
- Land softly back into a squat position.

6) Plank Jacks:

- Start in a plank position with your hands directly under your shoulders.
- Jump both feet out wide, then back together, keeping your core engaged.

Cool-down (2 minutes):

- Slowly walk or jog in place for 1 minute to bring your heart rate down.
- Perform static stretches targeting major muscle groups, holding each stretch for 15-30 seconds.

NO EQUIPMENT HIIT WORKOUT

Warm-up (3 minutes):

1. Jumping Jacks - 1 minute
2. Leg Swings (30 seconds for each leg)
3. High Knees - 1 minute

Main Workout (12 minutes):

Perform each exercise for 30-40 seconds at high intensity, followed by 1 minute of rest before moving on to the next exercise. Repeat for a total of 6 rounds.

1) Squat Jumps:

- Start in a squat position with feet shoulder-width apart.
- Explode up into a jump, reaching your arms overhead.
- Land softly back into a squat position.

2) Push-up to Rotation:

- Start in a plank position with your hands slightly wider than shoulder-width apart.
- Lower into a push-up.
- As you push back up, rotate your body to the side, extending one arm overhead.
- Return to the plank position and repeat on the other side.

3) Jump Rope (or Simulated Jump Rope):

- Perform as if using a jump rope, jumping lightly on the balls of your feet.
- Swing your arms as if turning a jump rope.

4) Reverse Lunges with Knee Drive:

- Start standing with feet hip-width apart.
- Step back with your left leg into a reverse lunge.
- As you come back to standing, drive your left knee up towards your

chest.
- Repeat on the other side, alternating legs.

5) Bicycle Crunches:

- Lie on your back with your hands behind your head, elbows out wide.
- Bring your knees towards your chest and lift your shoulder blades off the ground.
- Straighten your right leg while twisting your torso to bring your left elbow towards your right knee.
- Switch sides, bringing your right elbow towards your left knee in a bicycling motion.

6) Plank to Frogger:

- Start in a plank position with your hands directly under your shoulders.
- Jump your feet forward outside of your hands, landing in a deep squat position.
- Jump your feet back to the plank position.
- Repeat in a fluid motion.

Cool-down (2 minutes):

- Slowly walk or jog in place for 1 minute to bring your heart rate down.
- Perform static stretches targeting major muscle groups, holding each stretch for 15-30 seconds.

BIKE/STATIC BIKE/PELOTON HIIT WORKOUT
Warm-up (3 minutes):

1. Easy Pedaling (1 minute): Start with a light resistance and pedal at a comfortable pace to warm up your muscles.
2. Increasing Resistance (1 minute): Gradually increase the resistance on your bike and continue pedaling at a moderate pace.
3. Sprints (1 minute): Increase your pedaling speed to a moderate-to-fast pace, simulating a sprint without increasing the resistance too much.

Main Workout (15 minutes):

Perform each interval for 30-40 seconds at high intensity, followed by 1-2 minutes of rest between exercises, decrease resistance, and pedal at an easy pace to recover. Be creative and use any combination of the exercises below to complete 6 exercises total.

1) Sprint Intervals (30-40 seconds):

- Increase the resistance on your bike to a challenging level.
- Pedal as fast as you can for the specified duration, simulating a sprint.
- Focus on pushing and pulling with your legs to maximize power.

2) Hill Climbs (30-40 seconds):

- Increase the resistance to a high level, simulating a steep hill climb.
- Pedal at a moderate pace, focusing on maintaining consistent effort throughout the interval.

3) Speed Intervals (30-40 seconds):

- Decrease the resistance to a light level.
- Pedal as fast as you can while maintaining control and good form.

4) Resistance Intervals (30-40 seconds):

- Increase the resistance to a high level, simulating riding through rough terrain or against a strong headwind.
- Pedal at a moderate pace, focusing on maintaining a smooth and powerful pedal stroke.

5) Speed Intervals (30-40 seconds):

- Decrease the resistance to a light level.
- Pedal as fast as you can while maintaining control and good form.

6) Endurance Ride (30-40 seconds):

- Set the resistance to a moderate level.
- Pedal at a steady pace, focusing on endurance and consistency.

Cool-down (2 minutes):

- Easy Pedaling (2 minutes): Decrease the resistance and pedal at a comfortable pace to gradually bring your heart rate down.
- Stretching (2 minutes): Perform gentle stretches targeting the major muscle groups used during cycling, holding each stretch for 15-30 seconds.

Remember to adjust the resistance and intensity according to your fitness level, and listen to your body throughout the workout. Stay hydrated and have fun with your HIIT cycling session!

RUN/WALK HIIT WORKOUT

Warm-up (3 minutes):

1. Brisk Walk or Light Jog (1 minute): Start with a brisk walk or light jog to warm up your muscles and gradually increase your heart rate.
2. Dynamic Stretches (1 minute): Perform dynamic stretches such as leg swings, arm circles, and torso twists to further warm up your body and increase flexibility.
3. Increase Pace (1 minute): Increase your pace to a moderate jog or faster walk to prepare for the main workout.

Main Workout (15 minutes):

Perform each interval for 30-40 seconds at high intensity, followed by 1-2 minutes of rest between exercises. Be creative and use any combination of the exercises below to complete 6 exercises total.

1) Sprint (30-40 seconds):

- Sprint as fast as you can for the specified duration, whether you're running or walking at a brisk pace.
- Focus on using your arms and driving your knees high to maximize speed.

Rest (1-2 minutes): Slow down to a light jog or brisk walk to recover.

2) Hill Climbs (30-40 seconds):

- Find a hill or increase the incline on a treadmill.
- Powerfully walk or jog uphill, focusing on engaging your glutes and driving your knees forward.

Rest (1-2 minutes): Walk or jog downhill or on a flat surface to recover.

3) Interval Sprints (30-40 seconds):

- Alternate between short bursts of sprinting and walking or jogging recovery.
- Sprint for 10-15 seconds, then walk or jog for the remainder of the interval.

Rest (1-2 minutes): Walk or jog at a comfortable pace to recover.

4) Speed Intervals (30-40 seconds):

- Increase your pace to a fast run or brisk walk.
- Focus on maintaining a steady and consistent speed throughout the interval.

Rest (1-2 minutes): Slow down to a light jog or brisk walk to recover.

5) Endurance Run/Walk (30-40 seconds):

- Maintain a steady pace that challenges your endurance but allows you to sustain the effort for the entire interval.
- Focus on breathing deeply and maintaining good form.

Rest (1-2 minutes): Slow down to a light jog or brisk walk to recover.

6) Fartlek (30-40 seconds):

- Incorporate changes in speed and intensity throughout the interval.
- Alternate between short bursts of sprinting, jogging, and walking as desired.

Rest (1-2 minutes): Walk or jog at a comfortable pace to recover.
  Cool-down (2 minutes):

- Brisk Walk or Light Jog (2 minutes): Slowly decrease your pace to a comfortable walk or light jog to gradually lower your heart rate.
- Static Stretches (2 minutes): Perform static stretches targeting the major muscle groups used during running or walking, holding each stretch for 15-30 seconds.

Remember to listen to your body and adjust the intensity and pace according to your fitness level. Stay hydrated and have fun with your HIIT running or walking workout!

LOW-IMPACT MODIFICATIONS FOR BALANCE DISTURBANCES HITT WORKOUT

Warm-up (3 minutes):

1. March in Place (1 minute): Start with a gentle march in place, lifting your knees comfortably.
2. Arm Circles (1 minute): Stand tall and extend your arms to the sides. Rotate your arms in small circles, gradually increasing the size of the circles.
3. Side Leg Raises (1 minute): Hold onto a stable surface for support if needed. Lift one leg to the side, keeping it straight but not locked, then lower it back down. Alternate legs.

Main Workout (12 minutes):

Perform each exercise for 30-40 seconds at a moderate intensity, followed by 1-2 minutes of rest between exercises. Be creative and use any combination of the exercises below to complete 6 exercises total.

1) Seated Marching:

- Sit comfortably on a chair with your back straight and feet flat on

the floor.
- Lift one knee towards your chest, then lower it back down.
- Alternate legs in a marching motion.

2) Standing Leg Curls:

- Stand behind a chair or hold onto a stable surface for support.
- Bend one knee, bringing your heel towards your glutes, then lower it back down.
- Alternate legs in a controlled motion.

3) Standing Side Leg Raises:

- Stand behind a chair or hold onto a stable surface for support.
- Lift one leg out to the side, keeping it straight but not locked, then lower it back down.
- Alternate legs in a controlled motion.

4) Toe Taps:

- Stand behind a chair or hold onto a stable surface for support.
- Tap one foot out to the side, then return it to the starting position.
- Alternate legs in a controlled motion.

5) Seated Arm Circles:

- Sit comfortably on a chair with your back straight and feet flat on the floor.
- Extend your arms out to the sides at shoulder height.
- Rotate your arms in small circles, gradually increasing the size of the circles.

6) Seated Toe Taps:

- Sit comfortably on a chair with your back straight and feet flat on the floor.
- Lift one foot off the floor and tap your toes in front of you, then return it to the starting position.
- Alternate legs in a controlled motion.

Cool-down (2 minutes):

- Deep Breathing (2 minutes): Sit comfortably and take slow, deep breaths, focusing on relaxation and bringing your heart rate down.
- Gentle Stretching (2 minutes): Perform gentle stretches targeting major muscle groups, holding each stretch for 15-30 seconds.

Participants can take rests as needed throughout the workout, listening to their bodies and adjusting intensity accordingly. Hydration and proper form are important. Enjoy the workout!

4

Top 5 Foods to Stop

Refined Sugar/Artificial Sweeteners

Refined sugar, also known as white sugar or table sugar, is a highly processed carbohydrate made from sugar cane or sugar beet plants. The refining process involves extracting the juice from these plants and then purifying and crystallizing it to produce the final product, which is composed primarily of sucrose molecules. During refining, the natural impurities, such as plant fibers, vitamins, and minerals, are removed from the sugar juice, leaving behind pure sucrose crystals. While refined sugar adds sweetness to foods and drinks, it provides empty calories and lacks essential nutrients.

Refined sugar and artificial sweeteners can contribute to inflammation in the body through several mechanisms:

1. **Promotion of insulin resistance:** When we consume these sugars, they quickly enters the bloodstream, leading to a spike in blood sugar levels. In response, the pancreas releases insulin to help

cells take up glucose for energy. Over time, frequent consumption of sugar can lead to insulin resistance, where cells become less responsive to insulin signals. Insulin resistance is associated with chronic low-grade inflammation in the body, as it can lead to the release of pro-inflammatory cytokines and increased oxidative stress.

2. **Formation of advanced glycation end products (AGEs):** When sugar molecules in the bloodstream bind to proteins or fats without enzymatic control, they form advanced glycation end products (AGEs). AGEs can trigger inflammation by promoting the production of pro-inflammatory molecules and oxidative stress. Additionally, AGEs can accumulate in tissues over time and contribute to the development of chronic diseases such as diabetes, cardiovascular disease, and Alzheimer's disease.

3. **Disruption of gut microbiota:** These sugars can alter the composition and function of the gut microbiota, the community of microorganisms living in our digestive tract. Dysbiosis, or imbalance in the gut microbiota, has been linked to inflammation and various health conditions. Consuming excessive sugars/artificial sweeteners can promote the growth of harmful bacteria in the gut while reducing the abundance of beneficial bacteria, leading to inflammation and compromised gut health.

4. **Activation of the innate immune system:** Refined sugar consumption can trigger the activation of the innate immune system, our body's first line of defense against pathogens. This activation leads to the release of inflammatory mediators such as cytokines and chemokines, contributing to systemic inflammation. Chronic activation of the innate immune system due to excessive refined sugar intake can contribute to the development of inflammatory conditions and metabolic disorders.

Overall, while refined sugar may provide a quick source of energy, excessive consumption can lead to chronic low-grade inflammation in the body, which is linked to a range of health problems. Limiting intake of refined sugar and opting for whole, minimally processed foods can help reduce inflammation and promote overall health and well-being.

Therefore, it's recommended to limit intake of refined sugar and opt for healthier alternatives such as whole fruits, natural sweeteners like honey or maple syrup, or minimally processed sugars like stevia, raw cane sugar, or coconut sugar.

Wheat

In the 1950s, wheat underwent extensive crossbreeding as producers aimed to develop a high-yield, disease-resistant variety. By the 1970s, this hybridized wheat began spreading globally and was widely used in foods like pizza, pasta, and bread by the 1990s. This new wheat was introduced without any long-term safety studies to assess its potential health impacts.

Unlike traditional wheat varieties, hybridized wheat often contains higher levels of gluten and amylopectin A, a type of carbohydrate that can lead to rapid spikes in blood sugar levels upon consumption. These spikes trigger corresponding surges in insulin production, potentially contributing to insulin resistance over time. Furthermore, the altered composition of hybridized wheat may exacerbate inflammation in the body, which is closely linked to insulin resistance and the development of type 2 diabetes. Research suggests that individuals with diabetes (any type) or those predisposed to insulin resistance may experience greater difficulties in blood sugar regulation when consuming hybridized wheat products. Consequently, reducing or eliminating hybridized wheat from the diet may be beneficial for managing blood sugar levels and promoting overall health, particularly for those with metabolic conditions.

For individuals looking to avoid hybridized wheat and promote better blood sugar management, several alternative options are available. First, ancient grains like quinoa, amaranth, and farro offer nutritious alternatives to traditional wheat products. These grains are naturally lower in gluten and higher in fiber, which can help stabilize blood sugar levels and promote digestive health. Additionally, almond flour, coconut flour, and chickpea flour are gluten-free alternatives that can be used in baking and cooking to replace wheat flour. These flours provide added protein and healthy fats, further supporting blood sugar regulation. Incorporating more vegetables, legumes, and fruits into the diet can also help diversify carbohydrate sources while providing essential nutrients and antioxidants.

Table of Healthy Alternatives to Hybridized Wheat.

Hybridized Wheat	Healthy Alternatives (Low Glycemic Index)
White Bread	Ezekiel Bread, Sprouted Grain Bread, Spelt Bread, Rye Bread
White Pasta	Chickpea Pasta, Lentil Pasta,
White Flour Tortillas	Almond Flour Tortillas, Coconut Flour Tortillas
White Rice	Brown Rice, Basmati Rice, Wild Rice
Instant Oatmeal/Cereal	Steel-Cut Oats, Rolled Oats, Oat Bran
Crackers	Seed Crackers, Flaxseed Crackers, Sweet Potato Crackers
Pizza Crust	Cauliflower Pizza Crust, Portobello Mushroom Crust

Caffeine

Caffeine, though widely consumed for its stimulating effects, can have detrimental impacts on blood sugar regulation and cortisol levels, both of which play crucial roles in overall health. While moderate caffeine intake may have minimal effects on blood sugar levels for individuals with normal insulin function, excessive consumption can lead to significant fluctuations. Caffeine has been shown to impair insulin sensitivity, making cells less responsive to the hormone's signals and potentially elevating blood sugar levels. Moreover, caffeine can stimulate the release of adrenaline, a stress hormone, which prompts the liver to release stored glucose into the bloodstream, further contributing to spikes in blood sugar. This can be particularly problematic for individuals with diabetes or those predisposed to insulin resistance, as it may exacerbate glycemic control and increase the risk of complications.

In addition to its effects on blood sugar, caffeine can also impact cortisol levels, the body's primary stress hormone. Chronic consumption of caffeine has been linked to elevated cortisol levels, which can disrupt the body's natural stress response system and contribute to long-term health issues such as anxiety, insomnia, and metabolic dysfunction. Cortisol plays a crucial role in regulating blood sugar levels, particularly during times of stress, by mobilizing glucose from storage sites to provide energy for the body's fight-or-flight response. However, prolonged elevation of cortisol levels due to excessive caffeine intake can lead to insulin resistance and impaired glucose metabolism over time.

The maximum recommended daily intake of caffeine varies depending on individual tolerance levels and health status but is generally considered to be around 400 milligrams per day for most adults. However, it's essential to be mindful of other sources of caffeine, such as tea, energy drinks, and chocolate, as these can contribute to total caffeine intake. Additionally, individuals with diabetes or those prone to stress-related health issues may benefit from reducing or stopping caffeine consumption to support better blood sugar management and overall well-being. Avoiding caffeine is best!

Examples of caffeine-containing foods and drinks along with their approximate caffeine content in milligrams (mg):

Item	Caffeine Content (mg)
Coffee (8 oz brewed)	95-165
Espresso (1 oz)	63
Black Tea (8 oz brewed)	25-48
Green Tea (8 oz brewed)	25-29
Oolong Tea (8 oz brewed)	30-50
Matcha Tea (8 oz brewed)	70-130
Coca-Cola (12 oz can)	34
Pepsi (12 oz can)	38
Energy Drink (8 oz can)	80-300
Dark Chocolate (1 oz)	12
Milk Chocolate (1 oz)	6
Decaf Coffee (8 oz brewed)	2-5
Herbal Tea (8 oz brewed)	0

Dairy

Dairy products, particularly those derived from cow's milk, can be inflammatory for several reasons. One primary concern is the presence of certain proteins in dairy, such as casein and whey, which some individuals may have difficulty digesting. In sensitive individuals, consumption of dairy products can lead to an immune response, triggering inflammation in the body. Additionally, dairy products often contain high levels of saturated fats, which have been linked to inflammation and increased risk of chronic diseases like heart disease and diabetes. Furthermore, dairy products can also contribute to inflammation due to their potential to contain hormones and other bioactive compounds, as well as being a common source of food sensitivities or allergies in many individuals.

In terms of its impact on blood sugars, dairy products can vary widely in their glycemic index (GI) values. While some dairy products like plain yogurt or whole milk may have a lower GI, others such as sweetened yogurts or flavored milk can have a higher GI due to added sugars. Consuming dairy products with a higher GI can lead to rapid spikes in blood sugar levels, especially when consumed in large quantities or without balancing with other nutrients. Moreover, the effects of dairy proteins, particularly whey protein, may also influence blood sugar levels by stimulating insulin secretion.

Table listing healthy non-dairy alternatives:

Dairy Product	Non-Dairy Alternative
Milk	Almond milk, soy milk, oat milk, coconut milk, rice milk
Yogurt	Coconut yogurt, almond yogurt, soy yogurt, oat yogurt
Cheese	Nutritional yeast (for flavor), cashew cheese, almond cheese, soy cheese
Butter	Coconut oil, olive oil, avocado spread
Ice Cream	Coconut milk ice cream, almond milk ice cream, soy milk ice cream, banana nice cream (made from frozen bananas)
Cream	Coconut cream, cashew cream, soy cream, oat cream

These non-dairy alternatives can be used in cooking, and baking, or enjoyed on their own as substitutes for traditional dairy products. They offer a variety of flavors and textures while providing options for individuals with lactose intolerance, dairy allergies, or those choosing to follow a plant-based diet.

Margarine

Margarine has garnered criticism due to several factors that make it potentially harmful to health. One significant concern is its high trans fat content, which is formed during the process of hydrogenation used to solidify vegetable oils and create margarine's butter-like texture. Trans fats have been strongly linked to inflammation in the body, contributing to various chronic diseases like heart disease, diabetes, and obesity. Additionally, margarine's composition is notably similar to plastic, as it is just one molecule away from being classified as a plastic material. This structural similarity raises concerns about its effects on human health, particularly its potential to interfere with cellular function and contribute to inflammation and oxidative stress.

A healthier alternative to margarine is to opt for natural, minimally processed fats like olive oil, avocado oil, or coconut oil. These oils are rich in monounsaturated or polyunsaturated fats, which have been shown to have anti-inflammatory properties and offer various health benefits when consumed as part of a balanced diet. Additionally, using spreads made from nuts or seeds, such as almond or cashew butter, can provide healthy fats and nutrients without the harmful effects associated with trans fats found in margarine.

5

Top 5 Dietary Modifications to Stabilize Blood Sugars

High Fiber Foods

High-fiber foods tend to be low on the glycemic index (GI) for several reasons. Firstly, fiber slows down the digestion process, causing glucose to be released into the bloodstream at a slower rate, which helps prevent spikes in blood sugar levels. Soluble fiber, in particular, forms a gel-like substance in the digestive tract that slows the absorption of sugar, leading to a more gradual release of glucose. Additionally, high-fiber foods increase feelings of fullness and satiety, regulating appetite and preventing overeating, which contributes to more stable blood sugar levels.

Many high-fiber foods, such as legumes and beans, contain complex carbohydrates that take longer to break down into glucose compared to simple carbohydrates, resulting in a lower glycemic response. Diets high in fiber are also linked to improved insulin sensitivity, which helps maintain stable blood sugar levels. Furthermore, fiber acts as a prebiotic, feeding beneficial gut bacteria, and a healthy gut microbiome can influence the metabolism of carbohydrates and fats, contributing to more stable blood sugar levels.

Listed below are examples of healthy high-fiber foods:

- **Lentils** - Rich in both soluble and insoluble fiber, great for soups and salads.
- **Black Beans** - A versatile legume that's high in fiber and protein.
- **Chickpeas** - Also known as garbanzo beans, excellent in hummus and salads.
- **Quinoa** - A whole grain that's a complete protein and high in fiber.
- **Oats** - A great breakfast option, high in soluble fiber.
- **Chia Seeds** - Tiny seeds packed with fiber and omega-3 fatty acids.
- **Flaxseeds** - Another seed high in fiber and omega-3s, great for adding to smoothies and cereals.
- **Almonds** - A healthy snack that provides good fiber and healthy fats.
- **Avocados** - Unique for their high fiber and healthy fat content.
- **Broccoli** - A cruciferous vegetable rich in fiber and various vitamins.
- **Carrots** - Crunchy and high in fiber, great raw or cooked.
- **Sweet Potatoes** - High in fiber, especially when eaten with the skin.
- **Brussels Sprouts** - Another fiber-rich cruciferous vegetable, great roasted or steamed.
- **Leafy greens** - are rich in fiber and essential nutrients such as spinach, kale, collard greens, and arugula.
- **Pears/Apples** - Especially high in fiber when eaten with the skin.

Protein

Protein-rich foods tend to be low on the GI due to several factors. Firstly, proteins themselves do not contain carbohydrates, which are the primary macronutrient that directly influences blood sugar levels. Therefore, foods that are primarily protein-based, such as meats, poultry, fish, eggs, and tofu, have minimal impact on blood sugar levels.

Additionally, consuming protein-rich foods alongside carbohydrates can lower the overall glycemic response of a meal. Protein slows down the digestion and absorption of carbohydrates, leading to a more gradual release of glucose into the bloodstream. This helps prevent rapid spikes and crashes in blood sugar levels.

Moreover, high-protein foods often contain other nutrients, such as fats and fiber, that further contribute to stabilizing blood sugar levels. Fats slow down digestion and help increase satiety, while fiber adds bulk to meals and slows down the absorption of sugars.

Further research over the years has investigated the health benefits of animal versus plant proteins. One book that explores this in detail is "The China Study," authored by T. Colin Campbell and his son Thomas M. Campbell. This book examines the relationship between diet and disease, highlighting the benefits of plant-based diets over those rich in animal proteins. Based on extensive research conducted in China, the study found significant correlations between high consumption of animal-based foods and increased risks of chronic diseases such as heart disease, cancer, and diabetes. In contrast, diets rich in plant-based foods were associated with lower risks of these diseases and overall better health outcomes. The study suggests that animal proteins can promote cancer growth and other health issues, while plant proteins are linked to protective health benefits. The authors advocate for a diet centered around whole, plant-based foods to achieve optimal health and longevity.

Fats

Fats play a significant role in balancing blood sugar levels through several mechanisms:

1. **Slowing Digestion:** Fats slow down the digestion process, which means that carbohydrates are broken down and absorbed more gradually. This slower absorption rate helps prevent rapid spikes in blood sugar levels.
2. **Sustaining Satiety:** Fats increase feelings of fullness and satiety, reducing the likelihood of overeating and the subsequent sharp rises in blood sugar that can occur after consuming large amounts of carbohydrates.
3. **Reducing Glycemic Response:** When consumed with carbohydrates, fats can lower the overall glycemic response of a meal. This means that the combined effect of fats and carbohydrates leads to a slower and more steady release of glucose into the bloodstream.
4. **Enhancing Hormonal Regulation:** Healthy fats support the production and regulation of hormones, including insulin. Proper insulin function is crucial for maintaining balanced blood sugar levels.
5. **Providing Energy:** Fats serve as a long-lasting energy source. Unlike carbohydrates, which are quickly converted into glucose, fats provide a more sustained release of energy, which helps maintain stable blood sugar levels over time.

Incorporating healthy fats, such as those from avocados, nuts, seeds, olive oil, and fatty fish, into your diet can help regulate blood sugar levels and contribute to overall metabolic health.

Hydration

Chronic dehydration is a widespread issue affecting approximately 75% of Americans that can lead to various health problems, including fatigue, headaches, poor concentration, and more severe conditions such as kidney stones. Despite many people consuming hydrating beverages, this is often offset by the intake of caffeinated drinks, alcohol, and high-sodium diets, all of which can contribute to net fluid loss and dehydration.

Hydration is crucial for glucose control for several reasons. It helps maintain blood volume, which dilutes glucose concentration, aiding in better blood sugar management. Proper hydration supports kidney function, is essential for flushing out excess glucose through urine, and helps maintain electrolyte balance, which is vital for proper insulin function and cellular response. Dehydration can impair the kidneys' ability to remove excess sugar, causing blood sugar levels to rise by triggering the production of stress hormones like cortisol. Additionally, hydration is vital for overall metabolic processes, including carbohydrate metabolism, ensuring these processes function efficiently and contribute to better glucose control.

Drinking at least 64 ounces of water daily is important, but more is generally better. A good goal is to drink half your body weight in ounces of water while avoiding caffeinated beverages and high-sugar drinks such as juice, soda, and sports drinks. If you have a hard time drinking plain water, work on getting used to this by trying better options that are sweetened with stevia versus artificial sweeteners. You can also infuse fruit, or use lemon or lime to add flavor to your water.

Salt intake

Our cells need the proper minerals to stay well hydrated, in particular sodium and potassium channels in our cells allow fluids in and out. Iodized salt also known as "table salt" is known to cause fluid retention and pull fluid from cells causing edema. As our bodies are problem solvers they use more pressure to get fluid into cells, this is called hypertension or high blood pressure. Iodized salt only has about 3 minerals present, choosing an option like Celtic salt or pink Himalayan salt which both contain over 80+ minerals has increased benefits. All of these minerals are important for hydration along with glucose regulation as magnesium, calcium, and potassium are key in improving insulin sensitivity.

A simple way to begin incorporating healthy salt into your daily routine is to replace regular table salt with Celtic salt or Pink Himalayan salt. To avoid excessive salt intake, reduce consumption of processed foods such as canned and packaged items. For better hydration, add one granule of Celtic or Pink Himalayan salt (about the size of a sesame seed) to each 8 oz of water you drink.

Healthy Meal Recipe Ideas

"Eat Breakfast like a King"

Feel free to be generous with your servings of nutritious proteins and leafy greens; their fiber and protein content will help you stay satisfied for longer. Get creative with your choices—here are some of my personal favorites!

Avocado and Egg Breakfast Toast
Ingredients:

- 1 slice of spelt, rye, or sourdough bread (fiber)
- 1/2 ripe avocado (healthy fats, fiber)
- 1 large egg (protein)
- Optional toppings: cherry tomatoes, baby spinach, chia seeds, fresh garlic, Celtic/Pink Himalayan salt to taste, or a drizzle of olive oil

Instructions:

1. Toast the Bread: Toast the slice of spelt, rye, or sourdough bread until it's golden and crisp.
2. Prepare the Avocado: While the bread is toasting, cut the avocado in half and remove the pit. Scoop out the flesh into a bowl and mash it with a fork until smooth. Add a pinch of salt and pepper to taste.
3. Cook the Egg: You can prepare the egg according to your preference (poached, or scrambled).
4. Assemble the Toast: Spread the mashed avocado evenly over the toasted bread. Place the cooked egg on top of the avocado spread.
5. Add Optional Toppings: For extra nutrients and flavor

Nutritional Benefits:

- Fiber: Spelt, rye, and sourdough bread, along with avocado, provide dietary fiber, aiding in digestion and helping to keep you full.
- Protein: The egg offers high-quality protein, essential for muscle repair and growth.
- Healthy Fats: Avocado contains monounsaturated fats, which are good for heart health and help keep you satiated.

Berry Protein Smoothie

Ingredients:

- 1 cup coconut water
- 2 teaspoons hemp or pea protein powder (not whey)
- 2 teaspoons coconut milk
- 1 cup mixed berries (fresh or frozen)
- 1 tablespoon chia seeds or ground flaxseeds
- 1 handful of leafy greens (optional, such as spinach or kale)

Instructions:

1. Prepare Ingredients: Gather all the ingredients and measure them out.
2. Combine Liquids: In a blender, pour in the coconut water and add the coconut milk.
3. Add Protein Powder: Add the hemp or pea protein powder to the blender.
4. Add Berries: Add the mixed berries to the blender.
5. Add Seeds: Add the chia seeds or ground flaxseeds to the blender.
6. Optional Greens: If using leafy greens, add a handful to the blender.
7. Blend: Blend all the ingredients on high speed until smooth and creamy. If the smoothie is too thick, you can add a bit more coconut water to reach your desired consistency.
8. Serve: Pour the smoothie into a glass and enjoy immediately.

Nutritional Benefits:

- Hydration: Coconut water is hydrating and rich in electrolytes.
- Protein: Hemp or pea protein powder provides plant-based protein.
- Healthy Fats: Coconut milk and chia seeds or flaxseeds offer healthy fats.
- Fiber: Berries and seeds add fiber, aiding digestion and keeping you full.
- Vitamins and Minerals: Leafy greens (if added) and berries are packed with essential vitamins and minerals.

"Eat Lunch like a Queen"

Sometimes lunch may be similar in size to your breakfast as the Queen may eat just as much as the king. Make sure to fill this with healthy proteins, vegetables, seeds, and or nuts. Get creative, below are a few ideas to get you started.

Big Salad with Lemon Garlic Dressing

Ingredients:

Salad Base:

- Mixed greens (such as spinach, kale, arugula, or lettuce)
- Fresh vegetables (such as tomatoes, cucumbers, bell peppers, carrots, radishes, or red onions)
- Protein options (choose one or a combination):
- 1 cup cooked legumes (such as chickpeas, black beans, or lentils)
- 1 block tofu, cubed and lightly sautéed or grilled
- 1/4 cup nuts (such as almonds, walnuts, or cashews)
- 2 tablespoons seeds (such as sunflower seeds, pumpkin seeds, or chia seeds)

Dressing:

- 3 tablespoons olive oil
- 1 tablespoon fresh lemon juice (about half a lemon)
- 1 clove garlic, crushed
- 1/4 teaspoon salt (or to taste)
- 1 teaspoon dried or fresh herbs (such as basil, parsley, or oregano)

Instructions:

1. Prepare the Salad Base: Wash and dry the mixed greens and place them in a large salad bowl.
2. Chop or slice your chosen fresh vegetables and add them to the bowl.
3. Add your selected protein option(s) to the salad.
4. Make the Dressing: In a small jar or bowl, combine the olive oil,

fresh lemon juice, crushed garlic, and salt.

5. Add the herbs of your choice.
6. Shake the jar well or whisk the ingredients in the bowl until the dressing is well combined.
7. Drizzle the dressing over the salad.

Chickpea Salad with Cilantro

Ingredients:

- 1 can (15 ounces) chickpeas, drained and rinsed
- 1 cup cherry tomatoes, halved
- 1 small cucumber, diced
- 1/2 red bell pepper, diced
- 1/4 red onion, finely chopped
- 1/4 cup fresh cilantro, chopped
- 1 avocado, diced (optional)
- 2 tablespoons olive oil
- 1 tablespoon fresh lemon juice
- 1 clove garlic, minced
- 1/2 teaspoon ground cumin (optional)
- 1/4 teaspoon red pepper flakes (optional)

Instructions:

1. Prepare the Vegetables: In a large bowl, combine the drained and rinsed chickpeas, cherry tomatoes, cucumber, red bell pepper, and red onion.
2. Add the chopped fresh cilantro to the bowl.
3. Make the Dressing: In a small bowl, whisk together the olive oil, fresh lemon juice, minced garlic, salt, and pepper. If using, add the

ground cumin and red pepper flakes for extra flavor.

4. Assemble the Salad: Pour the dressing over the chickpea and vegetable mixture. Toss everything together gently to ensure the salad is well-coated with the dressing.
5. Add the Avocado (Optional)
6. Serve the salad immediately or let it sit in the refrigerator for about 30 minutes to allow the flavors to meld.

Customization Tips:

- Veggies: Feel free to add or substitute any vegetables you like, such as diced carrots, celery, or corn.
- Herbs: If you're not a fan of cilantro, you can use fresh parsley or basil instead.
- Extras: Add some crumbled feta cheese or chopped nuts for extra texture and flavor.

Customization Tips:

- Vegetables: Feel free to add or substitute any vegetables you like. Some great additions include avocado, beets, or roasted vegetables.
- Protein: Mix and match different proteins to keep the salad interesting and nutritious.
- Dressing: Adjust the seasoning in the dressing to suit your taste. Add a bit of honey or maple syrup for a touch of sweetness if desired.

"Eat Supper Like a Pauper"

Your supper is crucial for success, as it should be your lightest meal or even skipped in some cases. This approach allows you to reap the benefits of a longer fast and enjoy better sleep, as your food will be fully digested before bedtime. Here are a few ideas for a simple but tasty supper.

Vegetable Broth Soup

Ingredients:

- 4 cups vegetable broth
- 1 cup mixed vegetables (carrots, celery, onions, bell peppers, zucchini, etc., avoid potatoes), chopped.
- 2 cloves garlic, minced
- 1 teaspoon dried herbs (such as thyme, oregano, or parsley)

Instructions:

1. In a pot, bring the vegetable broth to a simmer over medium heat.
2. Add the mixed vegetables, minced garlic, and dried herbs to the pot.
3. Season with salt and pepper to taste.
4. Let the soup simmer for about 15-20 minutes, or until the vegetables are tender.
5. Serve hot and enjoy your simple and delicious vegetable broth soup!

Fresh Tomato Basil Soup

Ingredients:

- 2 tablespoons olive oil
- 1 onion, chopped
- 2 cloves garlic, minced
- 6-8 large tomatoes, diced
- 1 cup vegetable broth

- 1 teaspoon dried basil
- 1/2 teaspoon dried oregano
- Salt and pepper to taste
- 1/4 cup fresh basil leaves, chopped (for garnish)

Instructions:

1. Heat the olive oil in a large pot over medium heat. Add the chopped onion and cook until soft and translucent, about 5 minutes.
2. Add the minced garlic to the pot and cook for an additional minute until fragrant.
3. Add the diced fresh tomatoes to the pot. Stir to combine.
4. Pour in the vegetable broth. Stir well.
5. Add the dried basil, dried oregano, salt, and pepper to the pot. Stir to incorporate the seasonings.
6. Bring the soup to a simmer and let it cook for about 20–25 minutes, stirring occasionally, until the tomatoes have softened and the flavors have melded.
7. Taste the soup and adjust the seasoning if needed.
8. Using an immersion blender or transferring the soup to a blender in batches, blend until smooth and creamy.
9. Return the soup to the pot and heat through.
10. Serve hot, garnished with chopped fresh basil leaves.

6

Top 5 Glucose-Balancing Supplements & Herbs

Garlic

Garlic contains compounds like allicin and allylpropyl disulfide, which have been shown to have beneficial effects on blood sugar levels. These compounds help increase insulin sensitivity, allowing cells to better respond to insulin signals and use glucose from the bloodstream. Additionally, garlic has anti-inflammatory properties that may help reduce insulin resistance and improve overall blood sugar control. Including garlic in your diet can be a flavorful way to support better blood sugar management and promote overall health. Plus you can add garlic to just about any dish!

Chromium

Chromium is essential for maintaining optimal blood sugar control because it plays a crucial role in enhancing the action of insulin, the hormone responsible for regulating blood sugar levels. Chromium helps insulin function more efficiently by facilitating its binding to cells, which promotes glucose uptake from the bloodstream into cells for energy. Additionally, chromium helps stabilize blood sugar levels by improving the metabolism of carbohydrates, fats, and proteins. Research suggests that chromium supplementation may be particularly beneficial for individuals with insulin resistance (this can occur in ALL types of diabetes) or type 2 diabetes, as it can help improve insulin sensitivity and reduce blood sugar fluctuations. Incorporating chromium-rich foods or supplements into the diet can support better blood sugar control and overall metabolic health.

The recommended amount of chromium for diabetes varies depending on individual needs and health status. However, some studies suggest that chromium supplementation in the range of 200 to 1,000 micrograms per day may be beneficial for individuals with diabetes or insulin resistance. It's important to consult with a healthcare professional before starting any new supplement regimen, as they can provide personalized recommendations based on individual health needs and considerations.

When looking for a chromium supplement, it's essential to choose a high-quality product from a reputable manufacturer. Here are some tips for finding a good chromium supplement:

1. **Look for chromium picolinate**: Chromium picolinate is the most commonly studied form of chromium and is believed to be well-absorbed by the body.

2. **Check for third-party testing:** Choose supplements that have undergone third-party testing for quality, purity, and potency. Look for certifications from organizations like NSF International, USP, or ConsumerLab.

3. **Read the label:** Pay attention to the dosage and serving size to ensure you're getting the appropriate amount of chromium per

serving. Avoid supplements with unnecessary fillers, additives, or allergens.

4. **Consider your specific needs:** Depending on your health goals and preferences, you may prefer a standalone chromium supplement or a multivitamin/mineral supplement that includes chromium along with other essential nutrients.

Food Item	Serving Size	Chromium Content (micrograms per serving)
Broccoli	1 cup	11 mcg
Turkey Breast	3 oz	2 mcg
Green Beans	1 cup	2 mcg
Potatoes	1 medium	2 mcg
Beef	3 oz	2 mcg
Apples	1 medium	1 mcg
Bananas	1 medium	1 mcg
Spinach	1 cup	1 mcg

Magnesium

Magnesium is a vital mineral that plays a crucial role in a wide variety in many bodily functions, including muscle and nerve function, blood sugar regulation, and bone health. When it comes to diabetes and insulin sensitivity, magnesium's significance becomes particularly pronounced. Research suggests that magnesium plays a key role in insulin signaling pathways, facilitating the uptake of glucose into cells. Additionally, magnesium deficiency has been linked to insulin resistance, a condition where cells fail to respond to insulin effectively, leading to elevated blood sugar levels. Therefore, adequate magnesium intake is essential for maintaining optimal insulin sensitivity and reducing the risk of developing type 2 diabetes. Ensuring sufficient magnesium levels through dietary sources or supplements can be a valuable strategy in diabetes management and prevention, emphasizing the importance of this mineral in overall health and well-being.

Magnesium is used in nearly every function in our body and cells. That is why the signs and symptoms of magnesium deficiency can widely vary. Below are several examples of symptoms that can develop in magnesium deficiency:

- Muscle cramps or spasms
- Fatigue or weakness
- Nausea or vomiting
- Numbness or tingling
- Muscle tremors or twitching
- Difficulty sleeping or insomnia
- Irregular heartbeat or palpitations
- High blood pressure
- Poor circulation or cold extremities
- Constipation or irregular bowel movements
- Mood swings or irritability
- Anxiety or depression
- Loss of appetite
- Weakness or brittleness in bones
- Elevated blood sugar levels or insulin resistance

Here are some easy tips to help you find a good magnesium supplement:

1. **Check the form of magnesium:** There are various forms of magnesium supplements available, such as magnesium citrate, magnesium glycinate, magnesium oxide, and magnesium chloride, among others. Each form has its absorption rate and potential side effects. Magnesium citrate and magnesium glycinate are generally well-absorbed and tolerated with higher bioavailability.

2. **Look for quality brands:** Choose supplements from reputable brands known for their commitment to quality and safety. Look for third-party certifications such as USP (United States Pharmacopeia) or NSF International, which ensure that the product meets certain standards for purity and potency.

3. **Read the ingredient list:** Check the ingredient list for any additional additives, fillers, or allergens that you may want to avoid. Opt for supplements with minimal added ingredients.

4. **Consider your preferences:** Some people may prefer certain forms of magnesium over others based on factors like taste or ease of swallowing. For example, magnesium powder or liquid supplements can be mixed into beverages for easier consumption.

5. **Pro Tip:** Some high-quality combination magnesium supplements provide a variety of magnesium types, these tend to help improve more ailments that can be associated with magnesium deficiency. My favorite combination of magnesium contains Magnesium citrate, Magnesium glycinate, and Magnesium Malate.

Table of common healthy foods that are good sources of magnesium:

Food	Serving Size	Magnesium Content (mg)
Almonds	1 ounce (about 23 nuts)	80
Spinach (cooked)	1 cup	157
Cashews	1 ounce (about 18 nuts)	82
Pumpkin Seeds	1 ounce (about 85 seeds)	150
Avocado	1 medium avocado	58
Banana	1 medium banana	32
Dark Chocolate (70-85% cocoa)	1 ounce	64
Black Beans	1 cup cooked	120
Quinoa	1 cup cooked	118
Brown Rice	1 cup cooked	86
Yogurt (plain, low-fat)	1 cup	42
Salmon	3 ounces cooked	26

Note: The magnesium content provided is approximate and may vary slightly based on factors such as growing conditions and preparation methods.

Apple cider Vinegar

Apple cider vinegar (ACV) has gained attention for its potential benefits in managing diabetes. Some studies suggest that ACV may improve insulin sensitivity and lower blood sugar levels after meals, which can be particularly beneficial for individuals with diabetes. Incorporating ACV into daily life can be simple and versatile. One common method is to dilute 1 to 2 tablespoons of ACV in a glass of water and consume it before meals. It can also be used as a salad dressing ingredient or added to marinades, sauces, or beverages.

When choosing apple cider vinegar (ACV), it's important to look for one that is raw, unfiltered, and organic. Raw and unfiltered ACV contains the "mother," which is a colony of beneficial bacteria and enzymes that give ACV its characteristic cloudy appearance. The mother is believed to provide many of ACV's health benefits. Organic ACV is made from organic apples, which means it's free from synthetic pesticides and other chemicals.

Cinnamon

Cinnamon is a popular spice that has been studied for its potential benefits in managing diabetes and blood sugar levels. One of the key ways cinnamon may help is by improving insulin sensitivity. Insulin sensitivity refers to how effectively your cells respond to insulin, the hormone responsible for transporting glucose from the bloodstream into cells for energy. Research suggests that cinnamon may enhance insulin sensitivity, allowing cells to take up glucose more efficiently and thereby lowering blood sugar levels.

Additionally, cinnamon may also slow down the digestion of carbohydrates, which can help prevent spikes in blood sugar after meals. Some studies have shown that consuming cinnamon with carbohydrate-rich meals can reduce the rise in blood sugar levels.

It's important to note that while certain minerals, vitamins, and supplements show promise as a natural aid in managing blood sugar levels, it's not a substitute for diabetes medications or other treatments prescribed by healthcare professionals. Make sure to be working along with your healthcare provider.

7

Conclusion

And there you have it—my top recommendations to help you or a loved one manage diabetes naturally and effectively. I hope you found these tips and insights useful and inspiring, providing your body with the optimal environment to heal. Remember, managing diabetes is a journey, and incorporating these natural hacks can significantly enhance your overall health and well-being while improving your diabetes control. Your commitment to learning and making positive changes is truly commendable. Here's to a healthier, happier you!

If you found this book helpful, I would be grateful if you could leave a positive review on Amazon!

8

Resources

Archundia-Herrera, C., Macias-Cervantes, M., Ruiz-Muñoz, B., Vargas-Ortiz, K., Kornhauser, C., & Perez-Vazquez, V. (2017). Muscle irisin response to aerobic vs HIIT in overweight female adolescents. *Diabetology & Metabolic Syndrome*, 9(1). https://doi.org/10.1186/s13098-017-0302-5

Collier, R. (2013). Intermittent fasting: the science of going without. *CMAJ. Canadian Medical Association Journal*, 185(9), E363–E364. https://doi.org/10.1503/cmaj.109-4451

Gheflati, A., Bashiri, R., Ghadiri-Anari, A., Reza, J. Z., Kord, M. T., & Nadjarzadeh, A. (2019). The effect of apple vinegar consumption on glycemic indices, blood pressure, oxidative stress, and homocysteine in patients with type 2 diabetes and dyslipidemia: A randomized controlled clinical trial. *Clinical Nutrition ESPEN*, 33, 132–138. https://doi.org/10.1016/j.clnesp.2019.06.006

Guo, Z., Li, M., Cai, J., Gong, W., Liu, Y., & Liu, Z. (2023). Effect of High-Intensity Interval Training vs. Moderate-Intensity Continuous Training on Fat Loss and Cardiorespiratory Fitness in the Young and Middle-Aged a Systematic Review and Meta-Analysis. *International Journal of Environmental Research and Public Health/International Journal of Environmental Research and Public Health*, 20(6), 4741. https://doi.org /10.3390/ijerph20064741

Sapra, A., & Bhandari, P. (2023, June 21). *Diabetes*. StatPearls - NCBI Bookshelf. https://www.ncbi.nlm.nih.gov/books/NBK551501/#:~:text=I ntroduction,around%20250%20to%20300%20BC.

Southhampton SDA Church (2018, March 28). *Barbara O'Neill- Decoding Diabetes* [Video]. YouTube. Retrieved May 27, 2024, from https://www w.youtube.com/live/oPAYsx0qRl8?feature=shared

Viana, R. B., Naves, J. P. A., Coswig, V. S., De Lira, C. a. B., Steele, J., Fisher, J. P., & Gentil, P. (2019). Is interval training the magic bullet for fat loss? A systematic review and meta-analysis comparing moderate-intensity continuous training with high-intensity interval training (HIIT). *British Journal of Sports Medicine*, 53(10), 655–664. https://d oi.org/10.1136/bjsports-2018-099928

www.ingramcontent.com/pod-product-compliance
Lightning Source LLC
Chambersburg PA
CBHW072340270726
48659CB00022B/2098